Clear

The Complete Guide to Crohn's Disease & Ulcerative Colitis:

A Road Map to Long-Term Healing

Alexa Federico, NTP

Printed in the United States of America.

First Printing, 2017

ISBN-13: 978-1981952489
ISBN-10: 1981952489

Girl in Healing, LLC
P.O. Box 80362
345 Main Street
Stoneham, MA 02180

www.GirlinHealing.com

Disclaimer: The contents of this book are solely for informational purposes only and should not be used as professional medical advice. Consult with your doctor before making any changes to your regimen.

To Dr. Emonds,
This book would not exist without you. I am forever
grateful for everything you've done for me.

Alexa Federico

Table of Contents

—

Introduction

"Failure will never overtake me if my determination to succeed is strong enough."
- Og Mandino

By December 2007, I was a very sick twelve-year-old. Up until that point, my life was what most would consider normal of an American preteen girl. I had never been severely ill; the most sick I'd ever been was during a bout of the flu or stomach virus. I was on no prescriptions or supplements. I didn't get any extra vaccines outside of the basics. I had never broken or sprained a body part, not even an ear infection. And, if we want to go way back, I was delivered normally and breast-fed. I ate "healthy," in terms of what a lot of American families would call healthy. I loved fruit and ate some vegetables and wasn't picky about whatever meat was served with dinner. But I also had chips, cookies, ice cream, commercialized bread, and anything that would fall under "kid food." The stuff that comes out of laboratories and factories that no longer resembles whatever real food it was made from, if it was even made from a real food in the first place.

My health became a slippery slope slowly yet so quickly. It took a few months for me to completely deteriorate and reach a point of such illness that I have, gratefully, never reached again. The signs and symptoms started out small and built on each other. I didn't think much of them at first, but my parents sure did. I had mouth sores and knee pain and a decreased appetite. As I got worse, I was losing weight, having night sweats, abdominal pain after eating a few bites of food, random nausea and vomiting, and diarrhea.

Throughout this cascade, my parents brought me to my pediatrician's office repeatedly. My mom would point out my bony stature and ask why my nails were almost always blue. Would you believe me that the doctor dismissed us by saying I was just a skinny girl and this all seemed normal? That is exactly what happened.

We sought out more doctors and nurse practitioners who shooed me away without considering the possibilities. We had to have returned to that office six to eight times over a few months. Finally, one doctor suspected I had Crohn's. This was after my parents had brought me many times and I had physically gotten worse. From there, just a couple days after Christmas in 2007, I was referred to a pediatric gastroenterologist, a doctor who specializes in the gastrointestinal tract. That doctor was extremely concerned about my condition and suggested I be admitted to the hospital immediately. That night, my new journey began.

During a hospital admittance of about ten days, I went through multiple IVs, blood draws, x-rays and other imaging, and retold my story over and over to new doctors. After a two-day bowel rest of only drinking liquids, I ate cereal and milk, white bread, chicken fingers, and ice pops made of high fructose corn syrup and artificial dyes. I remember one day I even ordered ice cream and apple pie for dessert, which I promptly vomited back up while the other half was still on my plate. The final tests were a colonoscopy and endoscopy with biopsies that confirmed the hunch my medical team had: Crohn's disease. It's a chronic, autoimmune condition that does run in families, but the cause of the disease was unknown and there was no cure. I remember feeling a sense of relief that there was finally a name to what was wrong with me.

From there I followed what my doctors suggested to a T in hopes of feeling normal again. I was on Prednisone, Pentasa, Prevacid, and liquid iron (that tasted as bad as it sounds) that my dad had to wake me up to give me one hour before breakfast every morning. I followed their diet guidelines, which were not much at all. They said to stay away from whole grains, too much fiber, caffeine, and maybe dairy. Well I did that, all right. I still got to eat chicken fingers, bagels, chips, cookies, white bread, and milk and ice cream; I just got the lactose-free kind! The Prednisone kept me feeling good. My friends supported me throughout. Life wasn't *all* that different. That is, until I got sick again.

I made it past my one-year diagnosis anniversary, but just barely. I had tapered off the Prednisone and in February of the following year, I got as sick as I was the year before. I stayed in the hospital for a few days, received IV fluids, and got the okay to go back home. But in March, I had to be hospitalized again.

Since my first hospital stay, my parents were interested in what my diet should look like. I still remember a doctor mentioning the Specific Carbohydrate Diet (SCD) so briefly that it probably took him one breath to say it all. But with it he said there was no proof it worked and was very hard to stick to. His goal of discouraging us from that diet worked, and we went with his recommendation since he was the expert. But as I got sick again and again, my parents became more and more concerned that what I was living off of was making me sick. It made perfect sense to them, since this was a digestive illness.

We were at our wit's end when a solution was put in front of us. Relatives of mine had been seeing a doctor that we considered "alternative," as his approach is not the norm. I was resistant for sure, because I learned that if I followed his suggestions, I would likely have to give up *a lot* of foods I loved. Thankfully, my parents didn't listen to my pleas, and we went to meet with this doctor shortly after my third hospitalization that March.

I entered his office apprehensive and desperate. I left, for the first time, with empowerment. This man was so sure I would start to feel better. Honestly, I was not happy about all the foods I had to cut out, but I was willing to try it. I remember it was right before Easter that year. I had my last regular meal for the holiday (my family's homemade Italian pasta, sauce, and bread) and I then I started the new eating and supplementation plan the following Monday.

He was not wrong. In fact, I felt better within a couple of weeks at most. My transformation was miraculous. I couldn't believe I had done this myself. After tirelessly following the doctors' usual recommendations and hitting walls, simply changing what I was eating resulted in more progress in a couple of weeks than I had made in over a year.

In April of that year we had a family trip to Disney World planned, and we were all worried that I wouldn't be well enough to go. This new doctor believed I would be stable enough by then. He was right! We went to Disney and had a blast, and I was able to stick to my eating plan.

Since then, I have gone through so many life experiences and health challenges. Not only have I gone from pre-teen to teenager to a college graduate, but my mindset and physical health around my disease have radically transformed. Let me explain.

I held onto a lot of anger, anguish, and resentment against my body for many years. Looking back, I realized I misunderstood myself. I felt as though I was given a defective body. I thought I was dealt a rotten hand of cards and I would be living at a disadvantage my whole life. I proved myself wrong.

This is not to say my health is perfect. It's not. But that's not the point.

What I have written in the pages to come is meant to equip anyone with Crohn's disease or ulcerative colitis with empowerment they need to start making changes that they have control over for the sake of their physical, mental, and emotional health. I believe that there is not one way to heal. Health is your mood, thoughts, diet, energy, attitude, physical signs and symptoms, actions, reactions, happiness, and more. We cannot expect to reach optimal health by only addressing one problem. Every part of us works together, both the physical and the intangible.

My goal for this book is to have instilled a sense of strength in you. I hope you can come to see how much of your health is in your control.

And please, show yourself compassion every day. And love. Always love.

Disclaimer: *I am neither a medical doctor nor am I speaking about any individual cases of IBD. What's written in this book is information, not medical advice. Every person with IBD has an extremely unique situation and will respond differently to interventions. Always consult your doctor before making changes to your regimen.*

1. What is an Autoimmune Disease?

The human body is an intelligent organism. Everything it does is to protect itself and stay alive. When a substance enters the body that is not supposed to be there, the body knows and reacts. This is the immune system at work. Once the body detects an invader (called an antigen), antibodies are produced to destroy the invader whenever the immune system detects it.

In autoimmune disease, (auto-, meaning 'self' and immune, referring to the immune system) the immune system becomes chronically overactive and mistakes its own cells for those invading antigens. Over time, the damage from the immune system repeatedly attacking itself develops into a disease.

There is no known ultimate cause of autoimmune disease, and I do not believe there is one root cause, but several. Genetics contribute about 1/3 of a person's chance for developing autoimmune disease, according to Dr. Sarah Ballantyne.[1] Throughout this book I will be discussing factors outside of genetics that can be addressed, therefore decreasing the risk for autoimmune disease or improving symptoms of an established disease.

What is Inflammatory Bowel Disease?

Inflammatory Bowel Disease, or IBD for short, is a type of autoimmune disease rooted in the

---

15

gastrointestinal (GI) tract. The body attacks its own cells because it mistakes them for foreign cells that do not belong there. This constant battle in the body creates chronic (continuous) inflammation in the digestive tract.

According to the Crohn's & Colitis Foundation, "Recent research suggests hereditary, genetics, and/or environmental factors contribute to the development of Crohn's Disease."[2] In the following chapters, I will go over areas of lifestyle that should be addressed to live as optimally as possible with Crohn's disease or Ulcerative colitis.

The Differences Between Crohn's Disease, Ulcerative Colitis, and IBS

Crohn's disease is a form of IBD that can affect any part of the GI tract (mouth to anus), although the end of the small intestine (ileum) and the beginning of the colon are most often affected.

Ulcerative colitis only affects the large intestine (colon).

Irritable Bowel Syndrome (IBS) is not a form of IBD. IBS is not an autoimmune disease and does not cause chronic inflammation that leads to intestinal damage. However, IBS is still a health condition and should not be ignored. Diet and lifestyle factors should be addressed to improve health with IBS.[3]

Symptoms

Symptoms of Crohn's disease and ulcerative colitis range from digestive issues to problems in other parts of the body. A person with Crohn's or colitis may experience some or all of these symptoms:

- Diarrhea
- Constipation
- Stomach cramping
- Nausea
- Vomiting
- Joint pain
- Mouth sores
- Weight loss or gain
- Blood in stools
- Fever
- Fatigue
- Loss of menstrual cycle
- Night sweats
- Loss of appetite or feeling full easily

Testing

Before going to your doctor if you suspect you have IBD (or any illness for that matter) do your own research on the condition as well as the types of testing needed for diagnosis and come into your doctor's office with as much "proof" as possible. Document your signs and symptoms. A detailed log will provide a compelling reason for your doctor to go forward with tests.

A problem with IBD is that the symptoms are not always obviously Crohn's or colitis. GI issues are extremely common today and some of the most common symptoms like upset stomachs and abnormal bowel movements can be caused by a variety of things that are not autoimmune diseases.

Although doctors are giving autoimmune diseases more attention, potentially increasing the rate at which patients are being diagnosed, I want you to be prepared to stand up for yourself and your right to health. If a medical professional doesn't believe you have a condition serious enough to warrant tests, get a second opinion. Getting diagnosed in a timely manner will mean you can understand your body sooner and start healing faster. No one should suffer in silence because of one doctor's opinion. Nipping autoimmunity in the bud - in a sense - sooner rather than later can be the difference between a mild case and a severe case of disease.

Once your doctor is on board with testing and has physically examined you, he/she will likely want to do a blood test. Because in Crohn's and colitis the immune system is in a chronic inflammatory state, blood markers for inflammation like C-Reactive Protein (CRP) and Erythrocyte Sedimentation Rate (Sed Rate) will be higher than the normal ranges. Other markers may be tested like vitamin and mineral levels. Nutrient deficiencies are another nod to a diagnosis due to impaired absorption in the gut. I was diagnosed with iron deficiency anemia when I was diagnosed with Crohn's. This played a role in my extreme fatigue. Your doctor may also have a stool sample tested.

After a physical exam, blood tests, and stool tests, an endoscopy and colonoscopy with a biopsy is the gold standard for IBD diagnosis. You may be put under anesthesia or opt not to use it. I personally always choose it for my own comfort and decreased stress about the procedure (although these are routine procedures). Through the endoscopy, your doctor will use a scope that has a camera on it to view your upper GI tract and take pictures as well as take a biopsy (the removal of your intestinal tissue to be examined after the procedure). The doctor performs a colonoscopy through the rectum and takes images and biopsies of your colon and small intestine. It will be clear to the doctor where there is ulceration and inflammation, as well as if your condition is mild, moderate, or severe. The preparation for this is worse than the actual procedure! You will need to fast for a day and drink mostly clear liquids as well as drink a solution to flush everything out of your GI tract so the doctor is able to see and move the scope without food getting in the way. Your doctor may also want to do some sort of imaging, like an MRI, MRE, CT scan, and so on.

After all of this testing takes place, it will be time to make a plan with your doctor. The severity of your inflammation will be the foundation for the route you take. In subsequent chapters, I will overview several different healing methods. If you and your doctor decide on starting a medication, make sure they have taken you through the proper screening process. Some medications are not suitable for a small percentage of the population, and taking them could be very hazardous to your health. Of course, I am one of those people and so I am unable to take certain drugs because of it. I am glad my doctor checked, just in case, all those years ago!

These days, most medical offices and labs have online portals. I highly recommend you make an account. This is where any lab or test results will be posted. Be sure to keep track of all labs, tests, results, and any other information on your health history. If it's easier to keep hard copies all in one place, print out your results and keep them in a folder or binder. If you see multiple practitioners, I would give each a separate folder or keep different tabs for each practitioner in a binder. It might also be helpful to keep notes after visits with your doctor to remind yourself of what was discussed. If you ever change doctors, being able to review these notes will make the initial consult smoother when reviewing your medical history.

2. Having a Solid Support System

"The 'i' in illness is isolation, and the crucial letters in wellness are 'we.'"
– Unknown

One of the most difficult parts of having Crohn's or ulcerative colitis is that they are invisible illnesses. There have been plenty of times in my life when I have looked well on the outside, but that could not have been further from how I felt inside.

I've put on a façade to make it through middle school to college graduation, countless jobs, and social scenes.

To most people, you are going to appear just fine when the reality may be that your stomach pain is unbearable, you are exhausted from a night of unrelenting cramps, your joints hurt, and you have reached a new level of fatigue you didn't know was even possible.

There are going to be days like this; I won't lie to you and tell you that they don't exist. Do they still happen to me? Sure, but they are not my normal, thanks to the changes I have made in my life that promote healing. With an autoimmune disease, it's all about decreasing the bad days and increasing the good.

During these times, it's especially important to have supportive, understanding, and non-judgmental people around you when you're under physical and emotional stress. Your support system can make or break you.

I discourage anyone from trying to face IBD alone. Sure, only you can experience the physical symptoms. Only you have the final say in your treatment decisions. But this disease goes so far beyond that. It is not unreasonable to feel that the scope of Crohn's or colitis is too great to bear alone. I have certainly felt that way. Having a chronic illness is tough as it is, and trying to play the hero will only burn you out quickly.

Who's in Your Support System?

The people in your support system are your biggest cheerleaders. They may be significant others, siblings, parents, or other relatives. They may be coworkers, close friends, or people in your church community. It's not how you know them that matters most, but how they treat you when the going gets tough.

When you were diagnosed maybe they researched the disease. They ask you what it truly feels like to live with IBD in order to understand it better. Most importantly, they will understand when you need to cancel plans due to an unexpected flare or fatigue. They will never make you feel guilty for this. These people exist. You need to determine who they are and nurture those relationships. Let them know their love and concern means so much to you. Be grateful for them every day.

Detach from the Negatives

Sadly, not everyone in your pre-IBD life will have a healthy spot in your new life. There are always going to be "Negative Nellies" in the world and you don't need that! Here are some ways to detect those negative energy zappers in your life, although you will probably be keen on realizing them yourself:

- They question you or don't believe you when you say you aren't feeling well or are exhausted and may say, "You don't look sick."
- They do not believe that certain foods make you feel worse and might offer you those foods anyway. They might say something like, "A little bite won't kill you!"
- They make you feel guilty about cancelling plans. Unlike your supporters who assure you it's not a big deal and want you to rest, the Negatives will make you feel worse about missing plans.
- They seem to disappear after you are diagnosed.

By all means, you can and should explain to someone who is being a Negative how he/she is making you feel, especially if it's an important person in your life. Inform this person that your disease is an invisible illness. Let them know that their support and understanding during periods of hardship would mean the world to you when you are flaring. You could even send them information about your disease through email or in person, from sources such as medical websites and blogs. If they still do not understand, it is not your job to change the way they think. Do not feel guilty about not staying in touch with these people. Don't waste time trying to keep Negatives in your life who aren't willing to be there for you through the difficult times.

Healing is a complex issue and our emotional states surely play a role in whether we will heal or not. Unnecessary stress from others will only inhibit the healing process.

Where to Find Support

Even if you have incredibly supportive friends and family, you might be looking to connect with others who just get it because they have IBD themselves. I started to seek this kind of connectivity the summer before entering college. That's when I started an Instagram account documenting my meals. (This was way before I ever envisioned having a blog or pursuing a career in nutrition!)

Below is a list of websites that offer different ways to receive support. Whether you want to connect one-on-one, join a Q&A forum, or read other people's stories and more, these resources are a great place to start.

- The Crohn's & Colitis Foundation resources:
  - Find a Support Group
    - http://www.crohnscolitisfoundation.org/living-with-crohns-colitis/find-a-support-group/
  - Talk with an Information Specialist
    - http://www.crohnscolitisfoundation.org/living-with-crohns-colitis/talk-to-a-specialist/
  - Community page – Forums, Expert Q&A, Online Support Group
    - https://www.ccfacommunity.org
  - Support for Teens
    - http://www.justlikemeibd.org
  - Campus Connection for College Students
    - http://www.crohnscolitisfoundation.org/campus-connection/

- CrohnsandColitis.com
  - Advocate Program
    - https://www.crohnsandcolitis.com/advocate-program

- CrohnsDisease.com
  - https://crohnsdisease.com

- Public Facebook Pages
  - Crohn's & Colitis Foundation
    - https://www.facebook.com/ccfafb/

- CrohnsDisease (.com)
  - https://www.facebook.com/crohn sdiseasedotcom/
- Healthline: Living with Crohn's disease
  - https://www.facebook.com/Croh nsDiseaseHealthline/

- There are countless private Facebook groups for IBD and chronic illness. Just search using keywords such as the name of your disease.

- Join Instagram. The number of users on this social media platform is constantly growing, and that includes the number of health accounts! Before starting a blog, I had an anonymous Instagram account for years. I built many virtual friendships this way. Over the years we have lifted each other up during hard times, celebrated wins, and shared advice. I have met some of these people in real life and I hope to meet them all in person some day! Search for account names and hashtags using related keywords to find the people you want to connect with. Hashtags are like keywords with a '#' in front of them. Some examples to search are #Crohns #ulcerativecolitis and #autoimmunedisease, but the combinations are endless.

Facebook Group Tip: Feel free to join a bunch of

groups at first, but notice the quality of conversations going on. How do they make you feel? Are people sharing helpful tips, personal wins, and things you find inspirational? Or, do you scroll through negative talk and people dwelling on things that can't be controlled? Even though all groups start out with good intentions, sometimes people end up dropping in just to complain without adding any value. I have left several groups because of this. After feeling brought down by reading the posts too many times, I thought, "Why am I still here?" It's easy to forget you can remove yourself from online communities so quickly!

I want to stress this point: healing is much more than a physical process. Once you have accepted IBD, it's important not to dwell on "Why me?" Instead of focusing on what you can't change (the fact you have this illness now), focus on what you can change (what I'm talking about on these pages). Your healing will be limited if you do not move past the pity-party stage. We all do it; just don't make it your new life!

3. Conventional Medicine

"Good health care is a team effort between patient and doctor."
- Dr. Mark Hyman

Conventional medicine includes the classically-trained doctors and staff working in our hospitals. These may include gastroenterologists, primary care physicians, physician assistants, nurses, nutritionists, dietitians, imaging technicians, lab technicians and phlebotomists, and others working in our hospitals and medical offices. The majority of people will start here, as I did. Some people will choose to only utilize conventional medicine and others will test the waters outside the scope of western medicine. Everyone has their own beliefs on whether to follow one or many schools of thought, and everyone has the right to make their own decisions about what is best for them. I am not going to debate conventional versus alternative medicine here, but rather outline what to expect in each.

Finding the Right Doctor for You

"I don't like what I see," was one of the first things that "Dr. Sue" said to me at our first consultation. She said this while scanning my underweight body with her eyes. I felt like my chest had been stabbed with a dagger. I had such high hopes. After not seeing a

—
29

gastroenterologist for years because of past negative experiences, I went into this appointment with a positive outlook. I visualized having a wonderful relationship with this doctor who would be willing to work with me and become my confidant. The way the scene played out could not have happened further from my vision.

I had made the appointment in search of a gastroenterologist in order to get updated testing done. Of course, I was very much aware I was underweight, which was a driving factor to see a doctor. My gut might not always function correctly, but when it comes to that instinctive signal, it was correct in telling me that "Dr. Sue" was not going to be a good fit. I felt judged within minutes of meeting her. Not a good first impression.

Not all gastroenterologists think the same. Even a small group of gastroenterologists in the same hospital could have vastly different beliefs and ways of working with patients. There is nothing wrong with "shopping around" and not settling until you find a doctor who you feel comfortable with.

Some things to consider when you are looking for a gastroenterologist:

- Do you want to go with an older doctor who has more experience or someone younger who may have a fresher perspective? Newer doctors are often more up to date on the latest research and treatments.

- Are you more comfortable with a male or female doctor?
- Does the doctor specialize in IBD? Some gastroenterologists may specialize in IBD while others could be experts on the liver or other specific GI disorders.
- Does the doctor have a friendly, relatable personality? Or, is he/she cold, dismissive, or condescending?
- Does the doctor listen to your concerns, give you time to ask questions, and not make you feel silly about asking them?
- If you are interested in trying alternative types of medicine, does he/she have an open mind or set in their ways?

If you feel that a new doctor is not going to be a new fit right off the bat, like I did with "Dr. Sue," then you are under no obligation to remain a patient of theirs. As a person with a chronic illness, you want to foster relationships with doctors that you can trust for the long haul. When you feel comfortable with a doctor, it takes away the stress, anxiety, and overall uneasiness when it comes to going in for appointments, and it makes it easier to ask questions and voice your opinion. If you realize doctor is not meeting your expectations, you are still not obligated to stay with him/her, no matter how long you have been seeing them. The qualifications for finding the right doctor will differ from one person to the next. The most important thing is to be comfortable with the trust you put in your doctor.

To start the search for a gastroenterologist in your area, here are some tools:
- Crohn's and Colitis (.com)
  - https://www.crohnsandcolitis.com/find-a-gastroenterologist
- Crohn's & Colitis Foundation
  - http://www.crohnscolitisfoundation.org/living-with-crohns-colitis/find-a-doctor/

Medications

In general, there are five categories of medications your gastroenterologist may prescribe you.

- Aminosalicylates (5-ASAs)[4]
  - The purpose of this kind of drug is to decrease inflammation in ulcerative colitis and mild Crohn's disease.
  - Sometimes types also reduce inflammation in the joints.
  - Oral Aminosalicylates
    - Sulfasalazine (Azulfidine)
    - Mesalamine (Asacol, Pentasa, Lialda, Apriso, Delzicol)
    - Olsalazine (Dipentum) & Balsalazide (ColazalTM) for ulcerative colitis in particular
  - Suppositories

- Canasa
  - Enemas
    - Rowasa

- Corticosteroids (Steroids)[5]
  - The purpose of this kind of drug is to decrease inflammation. Most steroids are used for short periods of time to control flare-ups because they can cause more side effects if taken long term. They can be used alongside other medications for IBD or alone, as prescribed by your doctor.
  - Steroids stop the adrenal gland's production of cortisol entirely or cause it to produce cortisol very slowly. That is why tapering off gradually under the supervision of a doctor is critical.
  - It's important to be aware that steroids are immunosuppressive, which means the immune system's ability to fight off infection is decreased.

  - Oral Steroids
    - Prednisone (Deltasone) – This is the most commonly prescribed steroid. Two common side effects that Prednisone is known for among patients is weight gain (especially in the face, which people call "moon face") and

excessive hunger
- Methylprednisone (Medrol)
- Hydrocortisone (also available as an enema)
- Budesonide (Entocort EC & Uceris) - Entocort EC is for Crohn's and Uceris is for ulcerative colitis
- Enemas, Foams & Suppositories
  - Generally used for moderate to severe cases when oral steroids are not working
- Intravenously
  - Methylprednisone and hydrocortisone are available through IV treatment.
  - Generally used for severe IBD that cannot be controlled with oral or rectal medication

- Immune Modifiers (Immunomodulators)[6]
  - Immunomodulators also decrease the immune system's ability to function. Since it is the immune response that creates inflammation, that function is decreased, as well as the ability to fight infections.

o Immunomodulators are used when IBD symptoms cannot be controlled by aminosalicylates, antibiotics, or corticosteroids or due to other complications of IBD.

o While most conventional GI doctors will downplay the possible side effects, I encourage you to do the research and make an educated decision. These drugs have helped people reach remission who otherwise had a poor quality of life. That being said, each person considering an immunomodulator (and any drug for that matter), should make their decision knowing the purpose of the drug as well as possible side effects.

o Oral Immunomodulators
- Azothioprine (Imuran & Azasan)
- 6-mercaptopurine (6-MP & Purinethol)
- Methotrexate
- These drugs can take 3-6 months to work, so often steroids will be started in conjunction for quicker relief.

- Cyclosporine A (Sandimmune & Neoral) and Tacrolimus (Prograf) begin working one-to-two weeks after the regimen has started and are best for treating ulcerative colitis. Tacrolimus can also be applied topically.

- Antibiotics[7]
  - Most commonly antibiotics are used for treating infections like *Clostridium difficile* (C. diff), *Giardia lambia,* or other infections. Unfortunately, in eradicating the harmful bacteria, antibiotics kill off the useful gut flora as well. Probiotics are generally a good supplement to take for IBD and probiotics are especially important to replenish the gut flora when taking antibiotics.
  - Some common antibiotics used for IBD infections and occasional treatment:
    - Metronidazole (Flagyl)
    - Ciprofloxacin (Cipro)
    - Vancomycin (Vancocin)
    - Rifaximin (Xifaxan)
  - These antibiotics are given orally but in some circumstances may be given intravenously.
  - The side effects vary for each antibiotic from flushing to neuropathy to

tendonitis. As always, research the purposes and side effects of any drug you are going to consider. Do not be afraid to ask your doctor questions!

- Biologic Therapies (Biologics)
    - Biologic medications are another class of drug that is considered for people with IBD who cannot reach remission through other drugs or interventions. There are some serious side effects, although rare, that need to be contemplated.[8]

"Biologics are antibodies grown in the laboratory that stop certain proteins in the body from causing inflammation. Biologic therapies offer a distinct advantage in IBD treatment because their mechanisms of action are more precisely targeted to the factors responsible for IBD. For example, unlike corticosteroids, which affect the whole body and may produce major side effects, biologic agents act more selectively. These therapies are targeted to particular proteins that have already been proven to be involved in people with IBD."[9]

- Anti-Tumor Necrosis Factor Agents (anti-TNFs)
    - Improvements in symptoms vary and may take up to 8 weeks to see, although it could be sooner.
    - Adalimumbab (Humira)

- An injection (can be done yourself or someone else)
  - Cetolizumab pegol (Cimzia)
    - An injection (can be done by a nurse, yourself, or someone else)
  - Golimumab (Simponi)
    - An injection (can be done yourself or someone else)
  - Infliximab (Remicade)
    - Infusion that lasts 2-4 hours

- Integrin Inceptor Antagonists
  - Inhibits the inflammation-producing cells from leaving blood vessels and entering tissues.
  - Natalizumab (Tysabri)
    - For moderate to severe Crohn's in adults when other therapies did not work
    - Infusion usually once every four weeks
    - Important to consider that this drug can result in progressive multifocal leukoencephalopathy (PML), caused by an infection with the John Cunningham (JC) virus. You must be tested for the JC virus before starting Natalizumab. Your risk of PML is lower if you test negative for the JC virus.

- Vedolizumab (Entyvio)
    - For moderate to severe Crohn's or ulcerative colitis when other therapies did not work.
    - Thirty-minute infusion
    - Works only in the gut, unlike Natalizumab, which works throughout the whole body. Due to the localization of this medication it has not been shown to enter the brain.

Over-the-Counter Drugs

For the occasional need for immediate relief, some OTC drugs can be very helpful.

Pepto Bismol or Kaopectate are anti-diarrheal medications that can be very effective. I always keep Pepto-Bismol in my house in case a flare strikes. I also always take it with me when I travel. It's always better to be safe than sorry when you are not at home.

The main ingredient in these medications is bismuth subsalicylate. I was surprised when my environmental doctor suggested I try Pepto Bismol to help with my symptoms. I assumed that it was the type of medication that covers up the issue and the real cause of my symptoms would remain unaddressed. I was pleasantly surprised to learn that bismuth subsalicylate actually has medicinal properties.

In one study aiming to find successful treatments

to eradicate *Heliobacter pylori (H. pylori),* bismuth subsalicylate was shown to help eradicate the bacteria in 93.9% and 95.4% in the two groups that incorporated it. In the group that was not treated with bismuth subsalicylate, *H. pylori* was eradicated in just 64.7% of patients.[10]

Procedures

According to the Crohn's & Colitis Foundation at this time, they estimate that up to 75% of people with Crohn's disease and 23-45% of people with ulcerative colitis will need surgery.[11] According to the traditional way of treating IBD, doctors first manage the condition with prescription medications, and then surgery if all other drug therapies have been exhausted. Unfortunately, many doctors still don't consider helping their patients to change their diets or lifestyles, as I am explaining how to do here. Sometimes surgery is necessary to fix isolated issues, such as a blockage. But other times, surgeries provide permanent solutions such as removal of a colon.

The pitfall of surgeries is that they are not a permanent solution for health. Crohnsandcolitis.com states that symptoms reoccur in three years in 30% of Crohn's patients, and within 10 years, in up to 60% of patients.[12]

I am one of many who can say diet has changed my life for the better, and it actually saved me from needing surgery when I was severely ill. This is what fuels my mission to lay out all of the options that are available to you.

There are several types of surgeries for when medication and other interventions do not work. Below are the types of operations needed for different situations.

Strictureplasty

Strictures are when chronic inflammation in the gut cause the tissue to scar. This scarring is called a stricture. Strictures can lead to narrowing of the intestines. This is dangerous because less food is able to move through the intestines. During a strictureplasty, a surgery is performed to widen the intestines. No bowel is removed.[12]

Resection

When IBD cannot be controlled, the most inflamed parts of intestine can be removed during a resection surgery. Then, the remaining ends that were on either side of the removed area are joined back together.[12]

Colectomy or Proctocolectomy

A colectomy is the partial or entire removal of the colon. Traditionally, a colectomy is performed by surgically making an incision through the abdominal area. There is also a laparoscopic procedure. In this case, the necessary surgical instruments are inserted by small holes in the abdomen to remove the inflamed parts of the colon. There are many factors that will determine which way the surgery is performed, such as how much of the colon needs to be removed, the patient's age and health status, among others. The rectum may or may not need to be removed.[13]

A proctocolectomy is the removal of the colon and rectum. When these parts are removed, a new way to store and rid waste must be created. In a procedure called an ileostomy, the end of the small intestine that was attached to the colon is connected to a hole called a stoma. A bag attached to the outside will collect the waste. Self-maintenance is required to empty the bag and change it.[11]

Fecal Matter Transplant (FMT)

Fecal Matter Transplants (FMTs) or bacteriotherapy are fairly new as a treatment for IBD. They were originally being used for those with *C. difficile* colitis, but IBD patients may reap the benefits as well.

According to the peer-reviewed journal, Gastroenterology & Hepatology, twenty studies evaluating the effects of FMT on patients with Crohn's or Ulcerative colitis have been conducted. In a review of eighteen of these studies, 61% of Crohn's disease patients were found to have reached remission and 22% of UC patients reached remission.[14]

More recently in 2015, two studies were done, both on people with UC. The first group of 75 patients with UC was on immunosuppressant drugs and was given either weekly FMTs or a water enema. When reevaluated after seven weeks, the group given the FMT treatments was 25% more likely to achieve remission over the patients given water enemas (5%). The study also found that patients who received treatment and had been diagnosed with IBD less than a year saw greater results.[14]

Conversely, the second study showed a negative result. In this study, thirty-seven patients with UC went through two FMT treatments through nasoduodenal tubes or received a placebo. No notable differences were found between these two groups.[14]

It is worth noting, as the paper states, that the mode of treatment delivery could have impacted the very different success rates. Much more research has to be done for FMTs with IBD patients, but so far, this could be a promising treatment. Because this is a newer treatment for Crohn's and UC, this treatment may not be available in all states.[14]

Other Procedures

Other complications may develop that require action. These can be abscesses (bacterial infections that causes pus to develop into a boil that needs to be drained), fistulas (ulcers that connect to other parts of the intestine or organs and are treated by surgery),[11] and fissures. Fissures are tears in the anus, and are usually treated topically.

These are some of the most common medications and procedures used for IBD, but your doctor may discuss other options as well.

4. Alternative Medicine

*"Natural forces within us are the true healers of
disease."
- Hippocrates*

No longer does the phrase "alternative medicine"
bring a vision of something abnormal or socially
outcast.

Why should we even consider alternative
medicine, you might be asking yourself? If the United
States and other countries have the most advanced
technology at their fingertips and traditional medicals
studies are continuously being funded, why should we
try methods off the beaten path?

Here's why. Modern medicine focuses on is
silencing symptoms, not resolving the true cause of
what is producing those symptoms. What is
considered alternative medicine today is actually
tuning into our bodies to discover what needs
attention.

The human body is extremely intuitive. It
operates in a very specific way. The body knows when
something is wrong and it tries to fix it. Often, the
symptoms we experience is the body at work. The
body's ability to recognize an imbalance and attempt
to revive homeostasis (balance within) is called innate
intelligence.

We should be asking ourselves the most

—

important questions:

"Why is my body out of balance?
"How can I bring my body back into balance?"

Keeping an Open Mind

Anything unfamiliar to us is just that—unfamiliar. It's human nature to be curious at best, and skeptical at worst, about things that we don't know about. Take a look at how people in history have reacted to things they didn't understand. Usually, it was not in a positive way.

If you're considering alternative therapies, be conscious of your thoughts around them. When you read about acupuncture, are you instantly breeding negative thoughts? If a friend suggests essential oils, are you on the defense immediately, dismissing any positive effects people may have claimed? If so, pause right there. You are not in the proper mindset for trying something new. Negative feelings about something new could cloud the positive effects you may feel from it because you so strongly believe it won't work.

That being said, not every alternative therapy is going to work for you. One that works for you may make me feel worse. Just like prescriptions, some patients experience success, while others see no improvement or become unhealthier. That is because of bioindividuality; our bodies are genetically diverse and do not respond in the same way.

If you feel drawn to a new therapy, try it out! You shouldn't let other people's opinions of something prevent you from testing it, as long as you have done your research and it is safe. At least if it doesn't work out, you've eliminated one modality that will not be added to your healing protocol.

With Crohn's disease and ulcerative colitis, I highly suggest keeping a food journal at the beginning of your diagnosis, and using it as needed. I encourage you to use the same journal-keeping technique when you try a new therapy. Write down the date you started, how you feel before and after, and continue a general log of your symptoms. Often, healing occurs in small steps and you may not notice little improvements such as less stomach cramping or joint pain. On the other hand, if a new treatment is making you worse, keeping journal notes will help detect that, too.

Types of Alternative Medicine

These are just a handful of alternative therapies:

Acupuncture
Massage
Essential Oils
Sauna
Reiki
Physical Therapy
Biofeedback
Yoga
Tai Chi
Meditation
Herbal Medicine
Homeopathy
Therapy
Functional Medicine
Nutritional Therapy

Where to Find Alternative Medicine Practitioners

- American Academy of Environmental Medicine
  o aaemonline.org
- American Association of Naturopathic Physicians (N.D.s)
  o Naturopathic.org
- American College for Advancement in Medicine (M.D.s)
  o acam.org
- American Osteopathic Association (D.O.s)
  o Am-osteo-assn.org

- American Association of Acupuncture and Oriental Medicine
  - aaaomonline.org
- Nutritional Therapy Practitioners and Consultants (NTPs and NTCs)
  - nutritionaltherapy.com
- International Association of Reiki Professionals
  - iarp.org
- Re-Find Health
  - re-findhealth.com
- Paleo Physicians Network
  - paleophysiciansnetwork.com
- AIP (Autoimmune Paleo Protocol) Certified Coaches (these coaches also hold a base certification or licensure)
  - aipcertified.com/coach-directory
- American Institute of Homeopathy
  - homeopathyusa.org

For other types of practitioners, using Google or Yelp to search locally in your area should do the trick. Ask friends, family and co-workers. Often someone you know will be the bridge to a referral to a great practitioner. Another tip is to ask on Facebook; people love sharing their referrals there!

5. Self Care

"The part can never be well unless the whole is well."
- Plato

I spent a long time just focusing on my physical healing. The commitment to feel better, for me, was adherence to a diet free of the foods I knew would bring back symptoms. That helped, and still does to this day. But I learned that we are more than our physical bodies. We emit energy and our body and soul picks up on that. Our thoughts, words, emotions, and feelings contribute to the rise or decline of our health. Once I accepted that, I felt like I understood myself on a new level. It was scary but also relieving to know that my body understood me on cellular, emotional, and physical levels.

Do Things That Make You Happy

Doing things you want to do is a critical part of self care! Life is more than working. In fact, we have clearly overstepped our boundaries when it comes to work. Careers consume most people, and not in a good way. The answer to our biggest question as the human race–why are we on this earth–is most certainly not to slave away in careers that drain us and take away our joy. Sadly, most people aren't doing their true life's work, the stuff that makes their hearts sing. Overworking yourself in a job you don't absolutely love is stressful. Stress is a contributor to autoimmune flares and will make just about anything else you are going through, worse. Chronic stress leads to mental and physical burnout at best, and a debilitating flare-up at worst.

Can you think of a few things you actually like doing? Take out a pen and a piece of paper and write them down. You will probably remember some that you haven't done in a while because life has gotten in the way. Why not do those activities again? We can make excuses all we want about not having time, but in reality, we make a choice about every decision we make. Everyone has the same 24 hours each day. How is it that some people achieve so much success and happiness in those 24 hours? Now more than ever you need to start putting yourself first.

Some of my favorite self care activities are reading for pleasure, crocheting in the fall and winter (especially when I am making things as gifts), walking in nice weather, writing in a gratitude journal or just journaling my thoughts, cooking, getting a manicure/pedicure, and listening to music.

Schedule Things to Look Forward to

A habit that "keeps me going" is having plans scheduled. This tactic is especially helpful when you're experiencing a lot of symptoms and feeling down. For those of you in school or working jobs you don't take pleasure in, this will be of special use to you!

Personally, small things make me ridiculously happy. If you're not one of those people, train yourself to appreciate the "small" things. Put anything and everything on your calendar or planner. Some of these things could be family gatherings, meeting a friend for lunch you haven't seen in a while, having a chunk of time all to yourself, going for a nature walk, or trying a new restaurant.

We can quickly fall into a pessimistic mindset when we are physically and emotionally drained and overburdened. Having some positive experiences to look forward to will give you an extra boost to keep on going.

Say No

None of us want to appear sick, limp, or disabled. However, many of us know that when we don't look physically ill on the outside, people cannot see that we feel sick on the inside. We may be asked to go to parties, other social events, to work more (depending on how your career operates), or to pick up more responsibilities in other areas such as in your child's school.

These requests in themselves are usually innocent in nature. These wishes aren't a big deal until you are dealing with a flare-up. Because we are generally strapped for energy during these times (or for some, low energy is a daily occurrence), then these asked-for requests are too much to handle. What is important to remember is that you *always* come first, no matter what is being asked of you. If you are like me and don't want to disappoint people or let your illness get in the way of doing things, you will push yourself to meet these wishes. I am going to caution you against that. I have learned my lesson the hard way and I had to learn it many times before I believed it. Playing the hero will hurt you more than it will benefit the other person you are trying to please.

Release the Guilt

Unfortunately, it is possible you will encounter pushback when you decline these requests. Whether you tell someone you cannot commit because of your illness or whether you prefer to use a different reason, is entirely your choice. You are not even obligated to state why you can't commit to something. Your reasoning shouldn't matter because the person on the other end should accept no as no. I know it can be hard, but do not let a person guilt-trip you into changing your mind. They will be fine; you must focus on your health!

I have a blog post titled, Guilt & Chronic Illness, How to Help (or Help Someone Dealing) with Guilt (http://girlinhealing.com/guilt). Read this if you are dealing with chronic illness, or use this to educate family and friends who don't quite understand how you feel. There are several reasons why someone's response to you makes you feel guilty. Generally, they are not mad that you aren't saying yes to them. It likely goes deeper.

Sleep, Rest, & Relaxation

Sleep; like money, most people want more of it. Getting sufficient sleep will not only help you feel better day-to-day, such as giving you more energy, clearer thinking, and improved mood, but sleep also impacts your long-term health as well. In fact, getting less than six hours of sleep per night is related to chronic low-grade inflammation and insulin resistance, as well as a greater risk for obesity, type II diabetes, and cardiovascular disease.[15] So without plenty of sleep, we are keeping the chronic inflammation going even if we are attempting to decrease it in other ways.

People with autoimmune or chronic diseases often experience more fatigue than people without them. Someone once developed the "spoon theory" to explain what this is like. The theory says that a person with a chronic illness has a certain number of spoons each day. Each spoon represents energy. Some tasks require more spoons than others, but when they run out, so does your energy. I can personally relate to this. I have had days when I feel full of energy, so I take advantage of it and be productive. At some point, I hit a wall. I am either done doing much of anything for the rest of the day or I will need a serious chunk of time relaxing before I feel good again. If you have IBD, you must not overlook the power of sleep and rest. I recommend you pay closer attention to it than before you were diagnosed. This is one very important part of self-care that should not be ignored.

Tips for getting high quality sleep and sufficient sleep:
- Get to bed earlier! This seems overly simple, but how often do you say you want to get to bed at a certain time, but it ends up being much later? Maybe you found a movie you love on T.V., get wrapped up in a book, or scroll through your phone for hours. Set a time relative to when you wake up so that you can get a solid eight hours and stick to it.
- Get outside during the day. Getting sun exposure in the day tells your body that it is daytime. This helps to keep your sleep cycle on track, and by night your body will be producing melatonin to help you fall asleep.
- Turn off electronics before bed! Research shows that the greater the use of technology in the hour before going to bed is associated with greater difficulty in sleeping.[16] It's best to have technology completely out of the room.
- Make sure your bedroom is dark and quiet. Wear a sleeping mask, use earplugs, or put up

blackout shades if needed.

Sleep is when our body detoxes and repairs cells. That's one more reason why we must be diligent about our sleep!

Stress Management

We hear from everyone that we need to decrease our stress. Our relatives, doctors, and even the mainstream media are talking about the negative effects of stress. Stress not only affects our mood, but also our weight, hormone regulation, blood sugar balance, digestive health, and more. In fact, stress has been a known contributor to intestinal inflammation since at least the 1930s![17]

What is stress? It can be something such as experiencing extremely hot or cold temperature or running for your life from a bear. Stress can be tangible or not.

What is unique about stress is that it is subjective. Stress is more about how the situation is perceived by the person experiencing it more than the stressor itself.

An example of this is two people who lose their jobs. Person A is upset at first, but he knows he must move on to support his family. He updates his resume, seeks jobs in person and online daily, and reaches out to friends and family to be alert for any leads. He sees this as a chance to try something new.

Person B is outraged that he was let go. He felt he deserved a position after all of the years he put into his job. He stays home, not wanting to accept he was unemployed. Staying home day after day leads him to become depressed.

Do you see how two people can handle the exact same situation completely differently? We cannot always control the stressors in our lives (traffic, car accidents, deaths, etc.), although sometimes we can (leaving a job you hate, distancing yourself from negative people, asking for help, etc.), but we *can* control how we react to the stressors. That is where the power in taking control of your health lies.

Jamie Horrigan, a medical student with Crohn's and blogger behind SweetenedByNature.com knows firsthand how stress that goes uncontrolled can affect her IBD as she works through medical school.

"As a medical student with Crohn's disease, I know firsthand the importance of managing stress. Not only does stress make us feel horrible, it can also make us sicker. When we are chronically stressed, our adrenal glands release more of the hormone cortisol. Studies have shown that excess cortisol suppresses the immune system, compromises digestion and absorption, increases inflammation, and may lead to insulin resistance, metabolic syndrome, and various other chronic diseases. With IBD, it is extremely important to manage stress, as stress often leads to flares, debilitating fatigue, and increased symptoms.

Medical school is stressful as it is and even more complicated with a chronic illness. Many say medical school is like trying to drink from a fire hose, as the volume of material to learn in a short period of time is unbelievable. Additionally, our future residency placement is highly dependent on how well we perform on the board examinations. To stay well and help achieve my dream of becoming a physician, I focus much of my self-care on stress management.

When I am stressed, I go through this vicious cycle of not sleeping well, eating poorly, not exercising consistently, experiencing increased symptoms, losing productivity, and becoming even more stressed. During times of stress, especially exam weeks, I try to keep my daily routine the same, but it is also important to embrace change if the unexpected happens. A healthy routine for me includes eating paleo, keeping consistent sleep/wake cycles, exercising (even if it's a simple walk), socializing with family and friends, and taking breaks. My biggest advice is to listen to your body, take care of yourself, and rest. Remember, it's okay to say no. Finally, laugh and do something you love every single day, and you are well on your way to managing your stress."

A big takeaway from Jamie is that there is a known consequence when cortisol, our stress or "fight or flight" hormone, is elevated chronically. That's why it's crucial not to brush off stress as any less important than diet or medication. Do you see how Jamie's typical healthy routine involves a variety of lifestyle choices? She incorporates the right food and exercises for her, socializing, and even taking breaks and laughing! She knows from experience that a "deficiency" in these areas will make the scale unbalanced and therefore she makes time amid her demanding schedule for herself.

Sarah Choueiry Simkin also has Crohn's and is the blogger behind MyMindfulTable.com. Sarah uses these "five under five" techniques to manage stress and take time to align herself. The following excerpt explains five mindful practices that Sarah uses that can be done in under five minutes.

"I am a believer that managing your stress and showing care for your emotional wellbeing is more important the food you eat and the medication you take. Do not get me wrong, what we eat and what we put in our bodies in general is important but we often neglect how we feel mentally and emotionally.
"Below are five simple exercises you could catch me doing throughout the week and that I have found very helpful in managing my stress, keeping my spirits high, and allowing me to be present and process what I am going through.

- *4-6-7 breathing*
  - *This is an exercise you can do for one minute or five or more. I do this breathing exercise when my anxiety is very high and I need a way to help calm my body down. It is fairly simple. I breathe in for four counts, hold for six counts, and breathe out slowly for seven counts. The trick to is to keep*

my breath slow and steady, and to just focus on my breathing. This helps elicit the relaxation response in the body.

- *Gratitude*
  - *An oldie but a goodie. I like to start my day with saying three things I am grateful for. You can either write them down or say them in my head. I do this before I grab my phone and get lost in technology. The tip with this is when you say or write your gratitude, to really feel it. Feel the emotion of joy and happiness when you say you are grateful for your child or security and comfort when you say you are grateful for your bed. This exercise can take anywhere from one minute to two minutes. It's not very long but is a great way to start your day.*

- *Body Scan*
  - *This practice takes about five minutes and can take longer depending on how long you focus on each part of your body. You can do this lying down or sitting in a meditation position. Close your eyes and take five slow, deep breaths. Once done, start at the top of your head and check in with each area of your body as you scan down. Scan down every four inches or so and check in. You start with the tip*

of your head to your eyes, check in, and then send that area love and say 'thank you'. "Thank you to my brain for helping me function," "thank you to my eyes for letting me see those I love and everything around me," and so on, all the way down to your toes. To recap: You scan down four inches at a time. Check in. Say 'thank you' and show gratitude for each part of your body and what it does for you.

- o *If you happen to get stuck in an area that is in pain or has a lot of discomfort, stop there for an extra minute, place your hand there and send it love. Really create the feeling of love and envision sending it to that area. When it is tough for me to cultivate that feeling, I will literally visualize my stomach (for example) as a baby that I am holding and loving. This always helps reduce the discomfort and pain in that area.*

- *Affirmations*
  - o *I LOVE affirmations. My best advice for getting into affirmations and how to pick them out is by checking out Louise Hay. Her book "You Can Heal Your Life" and her website has helped me so much when I began to first venture into mindful practices to help heal my soul and body. You can use her app or website to help you create*

affirmations specific to what your needs are. One of my favorite and most simplistic affirmations I like to say or write in my journal for at least a minute a day, is "I am safe. I am whole. I am love." You can also write it down on a sticky note and place it on your bathroom mirror as a nice reminder that you are safe, whole, and love.

- *Simple Meditation*
  - *Simply 'being' at times is all we need. The permission to just sit and be. This can be very hard for many people, including myself. My favorite meditation to do is to sit still on my sofa, leaning back for support and keeping my back up straight. You can either plant your feet on the floor or sit criss-cross, whatever you are most comfortable in. Set your timer for one minute. Close your eyes. Take a big deep breath and just be. Focus on your breath. If thoughts come in let them go. Do not hold on to them but also do not exert too much energy to make them go away. You can start with one minute and increase it to five or ten minutes.*

o *This is a great exercise to do at any point in the day. The timer will also help take away that anxiety of "How much time have I been sitting here? How much longer do I need to sit here?" You can focus on your breath and not when this will end because you have a timer to let you know.*

I hope you all find these simple exercises helpful! Remember, doing one minute a day is better than none. Set your goals small, start simple, do something daily and work your way up. You will notice a huge difference in how you face stresses in your every day life and how quickly you can recover from emotional distress."

Stress management sounds like a lofty project, full of lifestyle overhauls and interventions. Yet, the act of rechanneling your perception of what is going on in your mind doesn't always have to mean *major* changes (unless of course, it does for you). When done with intention in a relaxed state, these quick practices can put you at ease and "reset" your mentality. Notice how you feel after implementing these strategies. Keep that feeling going as long as you can. When you notice your stress level start to get out of control, try to tap back into the calmness you felt before. I can confidently say at the very least you won't feel *worse* after practices like these.

6. Exercise

"The desire of activity is designed by nature to promote our physical well-being. Physical activity is the law of physical health."
- Edward Brooks

Benefits of Moving

For years I avoided exercise for two reasons.

Since I have been underweight for almost all of my life that I have had Crohn's disease (half of my life now), I thought that exercising would be detrimental to my recovery. Moving my body, which would burn calories and make me even thinner, seemed like the opposite of what was best for me, I thought. Even without moving regularly and eating a diet fit to my needs, I had struggled to put weight on and keep it on. I was *always* trying to put on weight.

The second reason I avoided exercise was because I just didn't feel like moving more than I needed to most days. Especially in the cold dark months of winter when I often feel worse, nothing about exercising appealed to me. My energy was unpredictable and I didn't want to "waste" it just to work out, and for what? I didn't want to get skinnier and I didn't care about building abs or muscles. Exercise just wasn't for my lifestyle, or so I thought.

In the spring of 2017, a decade since I was diagnosed with Crohn's disease, I was fed up with not feeling and looking the way I wanted to. I took pictures one day in my workout clothes and actually told myself that someday in the near future I would have healthier pictures to compare these to. I still have those photos on my phone.

One major change I made to my lifestyle was exercising. With the recommendation of a few friends and learning the valuable benefits of movement in my education through the Nutritional Therapy Association, I realized exercise was for everyone, not just for people trying to get thin. I did free online yoga videos a few times a week and a short, easy exercise regimen I got from a popular online fitness website that I found from an online search. In a few months I could see my body had been transformed. For the first time, I was happy with my weight. I'm not always motivated to move, and there are days where I don't. But understanding where movement fits into my health was a major mindset shift that I needed to go a step further in my healing journey.

One major benefit of exercise that is especially important for people with IBD is building and retaining bone mineral density. People with Crohn's and colitis are at a 40-50% risk of osteopenia (low bone mineral density) and a 26-30% risk of osteoporosis (severe bone loss/brittle bones).[18] These are conditions that tend to affect the elderly, but it's possible that even young children with IBD can experience extreme loss of bone density. Nutrient deficiencies, corticosteroids, and inflammation are potential contributors to a loss of bone mineral density that IBD patients can develop. In steroid use in particular, studies show that these medications contribute to fracture risk, muscle loss, and loss of endurance.[18] However, exercises like resistance training and aerobic exercise may offset these effects!

It's possible that exercise can play a role in preventing IBD in the first place. Interestingly, a German study that compared the incidence of IBD in men and women in various occupations showed that those working in careers that made them move physically and were outdoors had a decreased risk of developing IBD than those working in indoor offices.[19] This study aimed to find out why IBD was affecting people in higher socioeconomic classes more than any other group. It's yet another reason to take frequent walks and eat lunch outside (if possible) if you work indoors all day.

In a world where we have become more sedentary than active, studies such as these offer hope in a time when people have become chronically sick. Physical activity is one more piece to the puzzle that is in *your* control. You get to decide how you move and when you move.

Types of Movement for IBD

"Walking is mans' best medicine."
- Hippocrates

While exercise can be beneficial to the way you feel, or even life changing, choosing the right kind of exercise is important. Even in healthy individuals, high intensity activity can cause GI distress, like in "runner's diarrhea." Additionally, due to the fatigue many people with Crohn's or colitis experience, over exercising can contribute to burn out and affect your ability to have a productive day.

Personally, I enjoy walking and yoga the most. They feel relaxing and restorative and I get all the benefits of moving my body. More often, I feel energized and not overworked. Occasionally I will follow a short workout involving some small weights. Recreational bicycle riding is something I enjoy as well.

Baska and colleagues hypothesized that during exercise, some substances like bile, bacteria, and pancreatic secretions are able to pass through the tight junctions of the small intestine (which is the same type of activity that happens in leaky gut syndrome, but with undigested food particles), which the researchers attributed to the result of GI symptoms.[18] Researchers determined the level of intestinal permeability through the lactulose-to-rhamnose ratio method and found an increase of this ratio "...at 80% aerobic capacity peak exercise," which supported the original hypothesis

—

that strenuous exercise increased intestinal permeability. However, when researchers looked at the lactulose-to-rhamnose ratio method at 40% peak aerobic capacity (low-intensity activity), there was no evidence of an increase in this ratio.[18]

What does this mean? Well, for people already in a GI-compromised state and that are also likely to have leaky gut syndrome, high intensity activities may be problematic.

If you are an avid runner, CrossFit enthusiast, or an intense athlete of some kind and don't want to give it up, there are some things to consider. If you are flaring, notice symptoms daily, if your IBD impacts your ability to live normally while high intensity workouts are in your routine, I would strongly consider reevaluating your workout regimen. If the choice is between doing something you enjoy, or sacrificing your health, I believe that your health should come first. It's possible that if you take a break, work on more restorative exercise, and healing form the inside out that you will be able to incorporate it back in moderately.

If you are doing great while embracing intense physical activity, then you might be healthy enough for it. Always listen to what your body tells you. Being extremely exhausted after working out or seeing exacerbated IBD symptoms are definitely things to look out for.

7. Supplements

Bioindividuality

A common question people with Crohn's and colitis want the answer to is what supplements and vitamins they should be on. It's a great question, but there is no quick answer. Every human being has a different genetic makeup and a diverse medical history and therefore, will require different supplements. There is not a one-size-fits-all approach to vitamins and supplements, but there are common nutrient deficiencies that occur with IBD and supplements that have shown to help. Of course, our everyday diets also affect our nutrient status.

Before trying any new supplement or vitamin, you should **always** talk to your doctor or health practitioner to make sure it's the right one for you and will not interfere with medications.

Common Deficiencies

Our digestive tract, mainly the small intestine, is responsible for absorbing the nutrients we get through food so we can utilize them in bodily processes to stay alive. You know now that IBD is based in the gut. Inflammation in the GI tract will inhibit the body's ability to absorb these nutrients, which can lead to micronutrient deficiencies. We may also be losing out on nutrients through diarrhea or simply a decrease in food intake due to loss of appetite or the fear of causing pain from eating. Some drug therapies for IBD can also prevent the absorption of some nutrients.

There is clinical evidence to support reduced micronutrient uptake in patients with IBD. Vitamin A, vitamin D, and zinc were three micronutrients found to be deficient in a group of children diagnosed with IBD between the ages of 1-18 years old. A few patients also had a vitamin E deficiency.[20]

The Crohn's and Colitis Foundation recommends supplementing with calcium, vitamin B12, vitamin B6, vitamin D, folate, magnesium, iron and zinc as well as taking a multivitamin.[21]

Micronutrient deficiencies can present themselves in a wide array of symptoms. Anemia, which can be caused by several issues such as iron deficiency, deficiency of folate or vitamin B12, drug therapies, and chronic inflammation, is one of the most common complications of IBD.[22]

It's best to decide with your doctor what vitamins and minerals you need to supplement with. Getting semi-regular blood tests will help you keep on track of levels getting low, so that you aren't taking a shot in the dark and supplementing with whatever seems popular in the market.

Quality Matters

I wish taking supplements were as simple as walking into your local grocery or drugstore, choosing whatever vitamins you need, and getting started. Unfortunately, many of these common brands of vitamins and supplements don't use high-quality versions of whatever supplement they are manufacturing. Often, they are synthetic, but you can't tell that from the bottle. The body cannot absorb or will poorly absorb low-quality or synthetic vitamins. Even though you think you are getting a dose of something every day, your body is mostly likely not absorbing some or all, of that vitamin.

While supplementation is necessary for many people, incorporating whole foods that are nutrient-dense in vitamins and minerals is essential. Our bodies run on food for fuel, growth, and repair, so why not provide it with the best possible foundation?

Herbal Supplements

Ali Le Vere holds dual B.S. degrees in Human Biology and Psychology and is a candidate for receiving her M.S. in Human Nutrition in Functional Medicine and has done the research to bring less common, but effective healing modalities to light. Ali faces many autoimmune diseases and has taken responsibility for her own health. She is always sharing riveting research on her blog EmpoweredAutoimmune.com and as a Senior

—

Researcher and Staff Writer for GreenMedInfo.com. Below is her research on herbs that may be beneficial for IBD. As always, discuss any supplement you are interested in using with your doctor first.

Due to the deleterious side effects of allopathic treatments for inflammatory bowel disease (IBD), up to half of patients seek alternative options.[23] In addition to foundational approaches, such as an anti-inflammatory elimination diet, [24] establishing a balance of omega-3 to omega-6 fatty acids, [25] and optimizing vitamin D levels, [26] all of which are proven to ameliorate symptoms in IBD and attenuate disease severity, the following herbal remedies have empirical support in the scientific literature and may be options to explore with a licensed functional medicine physician. Synthetic medicines represent foreign, xenobiotic compounds unrecognizable by the human body, which disrupt the finely-orchestrated physiological symphony, whereas botanical medicines are biocompatible and have immense therapeutic potential when used as a complement to conventional therapies.

Boswellia

There is evidence that the staple of traditional Ayurvedic medicine known as Boswellia serrata, *or Indian frankincense, may be effective in Crohn's disease. Chemical constituents within Boswellia that elicit*

---

therapeutic activity include pentacyclic triterpenes such as 11-keto-β-boswellic acid (KBA) and acetyl-11-keto-β-boswellic acid (AKBA).[28] Not only does Boswellia decrease production of signaling molecules which perpetuate the pathophysiology of Crohn's disease, such as interleukin (IL)-1, IL-2, IL-4, IL-6, tumor necrosis factor (TNF)-α, and interferon (IFN)-γ, but it also inhibits synthesis of elastase, an enzyme, which degrades tissue, and reactive oxygen species (ROS), which contribute to the inflammatory burden. [27] Boswellia also suppresses a master transcription factor known as nuclear factor kappa beta (NFκB), which regulates production of pro-inflammatory eicosanoids such as leukotrienes, prostaglandins, and thromboxanes, which incite tissue damage.[27]

In fact, randomized controlled trials of Boswellia in patients with active Crohn's disease have shown that it has equal efficacy to a pharmaceutical standard of care known as mesalazine.[29] In another open-label study of ulcerative colitis patient in remission, a patented form of Boswellia significantly reduced levels of fecal calprotectin, a parameter of intestinal inflammation that is correlated with disease severity.[30] Boswellia significantly reduced all symptoms that were measured, including "diffuse intestinal pain, evident and occult blood in stools, bowel movements and cramps, watery stools, malaise, anemia, rectal involvement, number of white blood cells as well as need for concomitant drugs and medical attention." [30]

Wormwood

Use of wormwood, or Artemisia absinthium, dates back to ancient Egyptian and Greco-Islamic medicine. Although traditionally used as an anti-parasitic remedy, it was referred to as "a general remedy for all diseases" in medieval times given its therapeutic potency in a range of maladies. [31] Wormwood mirrors the actions of newer generation monoclonal antibody treatments such as infliximab (Remicade) and adalimumab (Humira) in that it targets and blocks TNF-α, without the concomitant side effects posed by these drugs such as risk of cancers, infections, and neurological complications. [32]

Patients with active Crohn's disease participated in a double-blind, randomized, placebo-controlled trial, where they received wormwood in addition to their regular doses of pharmaceutical drugs such as 5-aminosalicylic acid (5-ASA), azathioprine, or methotrexate. [33] During the study, all subjects were systematically tapered from steroids. [33] Despite being completely weaned off of steroids, 65% of those in the wormwood group attained near complete resolution of symptoms two months into the trial, which persisted throughout the five month period in which researchers observed subjects for any return of symptoms.[33] Wormwood elicited improvements in disease activity as well as in mood and quality of life (33). On the other hand, remission was not achieved in any subject in the placebo group, and the re-introduction of steroids was required in 80% of controls due to the progressive exacerbation of their symptoms.[33] α- and β-thujones, which are terpene-derivatives present in wormwood, carry attendant risks of seizures and neurotoxic effects at high doses, so they should not be dosed at greater than five parts per million.[34]

Turmeric

A long-time culinary centerpiece of Chinese, Iranian, Polynesian, Malaysian, Thai, and Indian cultures, turmeric is well-supported for a litany of chronic inflammatory and autoimmune disorders.[35] Although research has concentrated on curcumin as the active constituent of this golden-hued spice, other compounds within turmeric such as the aromatic tumerone may also confer healing properties. Studies have shown that curcumin may elicit immunosuppression by preventing the migration of white blood cells into tissue,[36] and by impeding activation of the pro-inflammatory transcription factor NFkB.[41]

When curcumin was administered to patients with Crohn's or colitis in an open label study, it reduced the inflammatory response in 80% of subjects, and moved biomarkers of inflammation such as erythrocyte sedimentation rate (ESR) and C-reactive protein (CRP) back into the normal range.[36] Some patients were even able to discontinue or reduce their dosages of 5-ASA or steroid therapy.[36] These results were replicated in a higher quality randomized, controlled, double-blind study of mild-to-moderate uncontrolled ulcerative colitis where curcumin induced clinical remission in over half of subjects compared to zero percent of subjects receiving placebo.[37] Although supplemental curcumin is often combined with black pepper, lecithin, or coconut oil for enhanced bioavailability, poorer-absorbed forms of turmeric may be preferable in IBD in order to prevent systemic absorption and to invoke local anti-inflammatory effects in the gastrointestinal tract.[38]

Aloe Vera

A drought-resistant succulent belonging to the lily family, aloe vera gel represents the leaf pulp of the Aloe barbadensis *Miller* plant.[23] It is a mucilaginous aqueous extract which has been used medicinally for millennia by the Chinese, Europeans, Indians, and Egyptians.[23] Due to its antioxidant, anti-inflammatory, and would *healing effects, it may have clinical applications for IBD. Aloe vera contains superoxide dismutase, an enzyme that constitutes one of our endogenous antioxidant defense systems which contributes to the neutralization of free radicals.[39] Its polysaccharides invoke various immunosuppressive effects, inhibiting an immune cascade known as complement[40] and reducing release of inflammatory mediators such as TNF-α, histamine, and leukotrienes.[23]*

When patients with moderately active ulcerative colitis were given aloe vera gel or placebo in a one month trial, aloe vera improved histological disease activity and produced clinical remission in over four times as many subjects compared to placebo.[23] Researchers in fact report that the magnitude of the clinical efficacy of aloe vera resembles that of mesalazine.[38] When subjects were scoped, the mucosal appearance of the sigmoid colon trended towards improvement with aloe vera.[23] Results may have been more impressive and reached statistical significance had the trial been larger; however, preliminary studies suggest that aloe vera may be a promising adjunctive treatment.

Resveratrol

Although wine is best known for its

resveratrol content, this phytonutrient can be obtained from foods such as grapes, blueberries, cranberries, coffee, chocolate, and peanuts. A polyphenol which has antioxidant, anti-inflammatory, anti-tumor, and immunomodulatory properties, resveratrol is being examined in pre-clinical studies as a potential treatment for ulcerative colitis.[44] Resveratrol enhances the expression of our antioxidant enzymes glutathione peroxidase (GSH-Px) and superoxide dismutase (SOD) in a concentration-dependent manner,[42] meaning that there is a linear relationship between our intake of resveratrol and our ability to neutralize the oxidative stress at the root of chronic inflammatory diseases such as Crohn's and colitis. In animal models, resveratrol up-regulates expression of anti-inflammatory signaling molecules such as IL-10, and reduces expression of inflammation-promoting enzymes such as prostaglandin E synthase-1 (PGES-1), cyclooxygenase-2 (COX-2) and inducible nitric oxide synthase (iNOS).[44]

Human studies are needed, but animal models show that resveratrol plays a protective role against the development of ulcerative colitis induced by a chemical known as dextran sodium sulfate (DSS).[43] When mice are administered resveratrol in tandem with DSS, colonic levels of SOD and GSH-Px significantly increase and the levels of inflammatory cytokines are markedly decreased.[43] Levels of colonic malondialdehyde (MDA), a surrogate marker for lipid peroxidation, or the oxidative stress-induced degradation of fats in cell membranes, which causes cellular damage, were also significantly decreased with the administration of resveratrol.[43] In another experiment, mice that received a diet enriched with resveratrol were protected against development of DSS-induced colitis.[44] The group that did not receive this prophylactic resveratrol treatment died at a rate of 40% after DSS was administered, while the entire resveratrol group survived.[44] Researchers state, "Our results demonstrated that resveratrol group significantly attenuated the clinical signs such as loss of body weight, diarrhea and rectal bleeding improving results from disease activity index and inflammatory score." [44]

Herbs that were used readily in the past are extremely underutilized today; despite the potent healing effects many of them carry. Unfortunately, Western medicine doesn't involve much if any education or training on using herbs. Additionally, although these herbs can be effective, they aren't very profitable because they cannot be patented into a drug like man-made medication can. If you are interested in using herbs, seek out an herbalist or someone such as a naturopathic doctor, who may be able to help you.

8. Environment

"Disease loads the gun, but environment pulls the trigger."
- Original Speaker Unknown

Your environment includes anything related to where and how you live. Some aspects of environment include living in a rural or urban area, medications, hygiene, physical activity, careers, stress levels, diet, child delivery, breastfeeding or formula-feeding, the products we use on our skin and in our homes, and pollution exposure. These are just some of the factors that shape our environment. With all of these conditions impacting our health, it's not surprising that our environment plays a role in disease prevention and treatment.

IBD is most prevalent in the most industrialized countries such as the U.S., Canada, and Western Europe. Interestingly, countries like India and China are seeing an increase in IBD as they become more industrialized.[45] This is a loud wake-up call, but it seems society just keeps hitting snooze. Ignoring these health problems will not make them go away, as we can see.

While we understand that factors outside of our genetics influence health and disease, the way in which these mechanisms interact with our DNA is not exactly known. Studies have been done on these various factors, but have mostly produced mixed results.

For example, smoking was found to be associated with increased flare-ups and need for surgery in Crohn's. Current smokers are at a higher risk for Crohn's disease then ex-smokers. This data has not shown true for Ulcerative colitis. Strangely, smoking has shown to have a sort of *protective* effect against UC. Those at greatest risk for UC are ex-smokers followed by nonsmokers.[45]

I want to make it clear I am not recommending anyone should smoke, as there are known detrimental consequences for smoking. This is just to highlight the discrepancies in the research and the need to invest more into studying how these factors influence IBD.

The study of environmental factors on disease is being looked at more closely. A 2009-2011 study observed heritable and non-heritable influences on the immune system using fraternal and identical twins as their participants. Researchers zoned in on 72 cell types in the blood to study and found that "...58% of all measurements having less than 20% of their total variance explained by heritable influences."[46] To summarize, more than half of the markers studied were overwhelmingly influenced by factors other than genetics. They did find a few cell types that were influenced more strongly by genetics, but concluded non-heritable influences were the majority.[46]

Studies like this one are great news for us. We, as well as our doctors, can lean away from blaming genetics and accepting a life of pain and misery and focus on the areas that have a *larger* influence on our immunity and that we can *control.* Even if you have already been diagnosed, working on improving your environment can only help your condition improve.

Doesn't that make you feel powerful?

9. Food

"Let food be thy medicine and medicine be thy food."
- Hippocrates

What's a cell in our body to think when we eat fake food? I'm talking about processed foods that are so far removed from their original source. It's not just the chips, cookies, and snack bars. Even most breads in the grocery store are overly processed and contain refined sugar, high-fructose corn syrup, and toxic oils. Have you looked at the ingredient labels in some conventional yogurts? Crackers? Frozen meals? This is "Frankenfood." When you don't recognize most ingredients on a label, that's a problem. As a modern-day society, we have altered our food so much that our bodies don't even recognize these food-like products as real food! Since having Crohn's or colitis puts us in a compromised state, we need to be extra diligent about the food we choose to nourish ourselves with.

Food is to gasoline as the human body is to a car. What happens when you put a really low-quality fuel into your engine? Sometimes you may get away with it, but eventually the engine is going to stop working optimally.

Our diets are a very personal part of our lives. Who wants to hear that their diet is unhealthy?

However, if you want to thrive despite having an autoimmune illness, you need to take responsibility where it's due and make changes in the areas you can control. Food is one of these.

Where to Start?

Cut out the Artificial and Processed Food

First, cut out the junk food. Get rid of anything refined or processed. Some of these ingredients include: food dyes, preservatives, refined sugar, high-fructose corn syrup, corn syrup, and refined "white" products like bread and crackers. You'll also want to avoid oils that have become rancid in their extraction and production such as: canola, soy, vegetable, corn, cottonseed, sunflower, and safflower oils.

Hopefully it goes without saying, but remove any conventionally-made chips, cookies, granola bars, cereals and other snack foods. Stay away from diet foods, which often remove fat and add in more sugar. This is the first step away from a SAD (Standard American Diet) and in the right direction of a diet based on real food.

Remove Food Intolerances

Keeping a food journal is the best way to determine what foods need to be taken out of your diet. There are plenty of food allergy tests on the market, but nothing is more reliable than your own sense of your body. I recommend logging what you eat and drink every day including medications, supplements, and vitamins and at what time. Also log symptoms and bowel movements with their times and how long and the quality of your sleep each night. Sometimes food intolerances can cause mood or emotional changes, so log these too!

Your food journal will become your database of research. Review it each day, and as you have more days filled in, i.e. more research to review, you will begin to see common threads. Did you have a terrible night's sleep after having ice cream for dessert? Maybe you noticed nausea after having a bagel for breakfast. These experiences will help you pinpoint what foods to eliminate (either temporarily or long-term). You could also start with one of the diets discussed in the coming pages.

The Big Offenders

"The incidence of CD has been increasing on a global scale, and it appears that is related to a "Western" lifestyle and diet, which shows the strong impact of the environment on the CD occurrence."[47] These findings are troubling and unless we take action, this upward trend will continue.

We have seen more illness over the years since we learned to refine foods and manipulate it in labs. We have come to the point where cheese puffs are a suitable snack but eggs are criticized for containing cholesterol. My philosophy when it comes to eating is to just eat real food in the most unprocessed state you can.

When it comes to autoimmune disease, some foods are consistently more problematic than others. Some of the most irritating foods are gluten, dairy, corn, soy, and refined sugar. I could go down the line and talk about other common food intolerances such as foods from the nightshade family (peppers, tomatoes, eggplant, white potatoes, and more), caffeine, or alcohol. For this section, I will go over why gluten is a major inflammatory food and why you see foods that are "gluten-free" labeled everywhere!

Gluten

Gluten is a protein found in some grains like wheat (and its many varieties), barley, rye, and spelt. If you're wondering why so many people are intolerant to gluten today when generation after generation before us ate gluten without any consequence, you are not alone.

There are several components to this question. First, our ancestors were not eating white bread or even the healthier-looking whole-grain wheat bread on your store's shelves. They made traditional sourdough bread that went through a lengthy fermentation process that broke down the gluten. This process pre-digested some of the gluten and made it easier to assimilate.

Next, our ancestors did not hybridize, genetically modify, or spray loads of toxic pesticides on their crops. The practice of modifying our food in labs or applying manmade chemicals is still fairly new in the grand scheme of time. Unfortunately, once these tactics were developed, they were implemented in full force without us knowing the long-term effects. The American population became the guinea pigs for these inventions to be tested on.

Gluten's Downfalls

Gluten contains lectins, a class of proteins usually found in the seed of plants. Some lectins can severely damage the gut and trigger an immune response.[48] These are meant to be a defense mechanism for the plant and the lectin will be indigestible to the animal eating it and/or makes the animal sick. Lectins can affect the rate at which gut cells are produced and are lost. They can also damage the cells in your gut lining as well as inhibit nutrient absorption, contribute to an imbalance of gut bacteria, and activate the immune system.[49] Not all lectins need to be feared and avoided. One type of harmful lectin is called prolamins. In gluten, the prolamin is called gliadin.

Zonulin, a protein made in the body, regulates the tight junctions in the intestinal wall, which means it determines whether the tight junctions in the intestinal wall are tight, which affects what passes through the gut into the bloodstream. Specifically, zonulin affects whether the tight junctions get loosened, which can let bigger, foreign particles through.[50]

We know that lectins have the ability to trigger the release of zonulin, which loosens the tight junctions and can move through the intestinal lining and into the body. This increases intestinal permeability (otherwise known as a leaky gut).[48] "Not surprisingly, increased intestinal permeability has been associated with autoimmune diseases... related to chronic inflammation like inflammatory bowel disease."[48]

Gluten-Free Diets and IBD

A survey-based study lead by the Crohn's and Colitis Foundation examined the connection between gluten-free diets (GFD) and IBD. They found that, "In this large group of patients with IBD, a substantial number had attempted a GFD, of whom the majority had some form of improvement in GI-symptoms."[51]

More than half of the 314 participants with IBD (65.6%) saw improvement in at least one symptom while on a gluten-free diet. Additionally, 38.3% of patients found they had fewer and less severe flare-ups, and 23.6% needed to rely on less medication due to a gluten-free diet."[51]

For someone eating gluten regularly, I understand how daunting it sounds to eliminate it. I didn't include this section just because it helped my Crohn's to improve, but because research like the studies I shared above is becoming more common, and the devastating implications of eating gluten with an autoimmune disease are being exposed.

Luckily, there is an abundance of resources to help you start going gluten-free. Blogs and medical websites are great places to start to find recipes and learn what to search for on ingredient labels.

Popular Diets

There are a number of diets people are seeing success with. I highly recommend keeping an open mind no matter what path you choose, whether you start with one of these diets, just go gluten-free, or start by just taking processed food out of your diet. Just because a protocol was tailored to resolve certain issues, doesn't mean it will work for you 100%. A food journal will come in handy here.

- Paleo & AIP
  - Paleo is known as the caveman diet. The purpose is to get back to real food, i.e. what our early ancestors ate before the cultivation of grains and legumes. This is not to be taken literally, because obviously we can't

all hunt for our own meat and seafood and grow bountiful produce gardens. Paleo excludes grains, legumes and refined sugar. Some say dairy or potatoes are not allowed, while others say grass-fed organic dairy and white potatoes are fine.

o AIP is a stricter form of Paleo structured as an elimination diet for anyone trying to heal from an autoimmune condition. The reasons these foods are excluded are backed up by science and have been found to cause leaky gut and inflammation. After a one-to-three-month period in the elimination phase, one will start to methodically introduce a food at a time, following the timeline provided.

o Visit autoimmunewellness.com and thepaleomom.com for two standout resources for the AIP and Paleo diets.

o The first study ever conducted on the AIP diet in 2017 included 15 patients with IBD who followed the "SAD to AIP in SIX" program created by Angie Alt.[52] The participants followed the elimination phase of the AIP diet for six weeks followed by a five-week maintenance period where no foods were reintroduced. The result? Out of the 15 participants, 11 achieved clinical remission by the sixth week (73%). During the maintenance period of five weeks, all 11 participants remained in remission.[52]

- SCD (Specific Carbohydrate Diet)
  - Elaine Gottschall wrote "Breaking the Vicious Cycle," which is a blueprint of the SCD diet. Elaine's daughter was extremely ill in the 1950's and was told, like many sick people still today, that diet had nothing to do with her unfixable symptoms and that she was destined to have her intestine taken out or die. The SCD diet is what one sole doctor guided her daughter through, and it saved her life.
  - The SCD diet eliminates hard-to-digest carbohydrates that will feed harmful bacteria when not broken down. The idea is that without these complex carbohydrates, the harmful bacteria have no food to eat and will not thrive. SCD excludes polysaccharides, disaccharides and includes monosaccharides and

fermented yogurt.
- o Visit breakingtheviciouscycle.info and read the book, Breaking the Vicious Cycle for more on the SCD diet.

- • GAPS
  - o GAPS stands for Gut and Psychology Syndrome and was developed by Dr. Natasha Campbell-McBride based on the SCD diet. It was developed to help people with digestive and psychological issues.
  - o The GAPS protocol is based on diet, supplementation, and detoxification. Like SCD, it eliminates hard-to-digest foods and includes an Introduction GAPS and a Full GAPS protocol. Depending on the health issues at hand, you may do both or skip to the full protocol. Dr. Campbell-McBride provides supplements that are generally helpful for people going through the program. Her view on detoxification is to aid the body's natural detox pathways gently to help damaged tissues repair and lighten the load the body has to carry.

- Visit gapsdiet.com and read Dr. Campbell-McBride's book, "Gut and Psychology Syndrome," for more on the GAPS diet.

- Wahl's Protocol
  - This protocol has a fascinating back-story. Dr. Terry Wahls, a doctor and researcher herself, was diagnosed with multiple sclerosis (MS) in 2000, after developing her first symptoms years before. She tried the medications that were available for MS, including chemotherapy, but her condition worsened and she was restricted to using a wheelchair. She did her own research on multiple sclerosis and discovered what vitamins and supplements were beneficial for MS and brain health and she was able to slow (but not stop) progression of her illness.
  - She came across the Institute for Functional Medicine after that and had the idea to get the nutrients she needed from her food rather than from isolated supplements. Started a combination of a paleo-type diet and neuromuscular electrical stimulation. This led to incredible

recovery. A year later she was able to walk again and do an 18-mile bicycle tour.

- o The Wahls Protocol is based heavily on nutrient-dense vegetables and fruits, but it is not a vegetarian diet. She recommends three cups of greens, three cups of sulfur-rich vegetables, and three cups of deeply pigmented fruits and vegetables per day! She also recommends eating 6-12 ounces of protein and plenty of omega-3 and omega-6 fats.
- o Visit TerryWahls.com and read her books, "The Wahls Protocol" and "The Wahls Protocol Cooking for Life" for more on the lifestyle program she developed for all chronic autoimmune conditions. She also has a practitioner training program for implementing the Wahl's Protocol.

- Low FODMAP
  - o FODMAP stands for: Fermentable Oligosaccharides Disaccharides Monosaccharides and Polyols. FODMAP foods

have carbohydrates (sugars) that commonly cause bloating, gas, or diarrhea in people who have trouble digesting them. Not all carbohydrates are FODMAP foods, so it's important to know which are and aren't in order to successfully try this diet.

o Therefore, the goal is to remove foods with FODMAPs and stick to few or no FODMAPs.

o Excluded are lactose from dairy, legumes, certain fruit and vegetables, wheat, and sugar alcohols.

o At the time I am writing this, SheCantEatWhat.com and KateScarlata.com are two fodmap-focused websites that provide an abundance of resources to follow this diet.

- Elemental Diet

o An elemental diet is an all-liquid diet. When IBD cannot be controlled and it seems all foods and causing problems, an all-liquid diet gives the digestive system a break.

o There are premade formulas on the market and I would

recommend researching what the ingredients are made from before choosing one. There are also recipes online to make your own.

o The elemental diet was shown to be as effective as Prednisone in newly diagnosed patients with Crohn's and previously diagnosed patients experiencing a flare-up.[53]

o Patient compliance is a major reason why this isn't recommended more, as the formula does not taste good. However, this is an option for people in acute situations.

Little Changes, Big Difference!

Relax

As efficient and miraculous as the human body is, it prioritizes dealing with the most urgent issue at hand. That's why when you are in danger—let's say a bear is chasing you and you trip and fall and have huge gashes in your legs and a twisted ankle–you are able to keep running and not notice how much pain you're in. Due to the surge in adrenaline, your body knows that survival is your number one concern, and it will focus on healing your wounds once you are out of danger.

The same goes for other bodily processes like digestion. Here's the plain and simple truth: digestion will not be effective if your body is in a sympathetic (stressed) state. You must be in a parasympathetic (relaxed) state to digest properly. So what does this mean? Most obviously, if you are doing any of the following while eating: doing work, arguing with your kids or spouse, driving, feeling nervous or anxious, or even watching an upsetting news story that has you riled up inside, then your digestion is impaired. Your body is also in a sympathetic state when you are standing. So eating over the sink or snacking at the refrigerator may be doing more damage than leaving crumbs on the floor.

Digestion starts when we first see our food. That registers in the brain, and the brain sends signals to the body to start preparing for digestion.

Slow down. Prepare your food. See it and smell it. Be grateful for it. Sit down, and *then* enjoy.

Chew

Once the brain and body are aware that food is going to be coming, saliva is produced along with the enzyme salivary amylase. This enzyme starts to break down carbohydrates while the food is being chewed up in your mouth. If you aren't chewing thoroughly, this first step in digestion is missed and you are already a step behind.

The truth is, most people chew each bite a few times at best, then swallow in order to get more food down the hatch as quickly as possible. On average, each bite needs 30 seconds or about 30 chews. Chewing food well goes hand-in-hand with eating in a relaxed manner.

10. Traveling

"The world is a book and those who do not travel read only one page."
- Saint Augustine of Hippo

Traveling with Crohn's or colitis is 100% doable, you just need to prepare in advance.

Where to?

Are you staying in a log cabin amidst the mountains? A resort? A relative's house? Where you stay is important to consider. Keep these questions in mind when planning, and then do some research about the area.

- Is there a grocery store nearby?
    - If yes, think about how you will get there. Are you driving to your destination? If flying, can your cab driver make a stop on the way to your destination? Can a family member drive you? Are there services like Uber and Lyft in the area? Maybe a grocery store has a delivery service and you can have food delivered to your destination.

- Will you be cooking for myself or eating meals prepared by someone else?
  - If eating at a hotel or restaurant, call them before you get there and explain what foods you avoid. Restaurants are so accommodating these days, so it should not be an issue, but it helps the kitchen staff out a lot to know you are coming in advance.
  - If you're saying with family, do your relatives know about your food sensitivities? If they are not well-versed with your eating style, let them know in advance that you are happy to help cook and bring some ingredients that you know will work for you. We can't expect hosts to do all the work themselves, so if we come prepared and ready to educate, as well as do the work, we make their lives a little easier.
  - This is where finding a grocery store comes in if you are traveling far and cannot take perishable foods with you. Always, always, take non-perishable snacks that you can travel with. They will definitely come in handy!

- Do I have access to bathrooms on the way there?
    - This is important if bathroom urgency is a symptom of yours. Of course, there are bathrooms in airplanes and trains. If urgency is an issue, it's wise to sit near the bathroom. If you are driving a long distance, make sure there are public bathrooms throughout your route you can stop in if needed.
    - If staying at a hostel, B&B, or Airbnb, find out if you have your own bathroom or if it's shared.

Travel Checklist

- Stash of emergency non-perishable safe snacks
- Perishable food if you can keep it cold in a cooler
- Pack more medication/supplements than you need, just in case
- Doctor/health practitioner's phone numbers/emails
- If driving, mapping out public restrooms to stop at if urgency strikes
- If flying or travelling by train, trying to get a seat near the bathrooms if urgency is a concern

- Calling ahead to hotels/resorts/Airbnb hosts to find out what grocery stores and restaurants are in the area
- Calling nearby restaurants (if eating out) to talk to the staff during off-hours to discuss if safe preparation of your food is possible
- Make a list of grocery stores and restaurants, and make reservations when possible
- Packing extra clothes (including comfortable clothing, shoes, and layers)
- Pack books, movies, journals, or other portable activities to bring if you are stuck inside not feeling well
- Heating pad

11. Getting Involved & Giving Back

"The power of community to create health is far greater than any physician, clinic or hospital."
- Dr. Mark Hyman

One of the best ways to empower yourself and others with IBD is to find a way to make your mark on the community you are now a part of. When you have that one thing, all of a sudden this disease has given you a new purpose.

Courtney Maiorino has Crohn's disease and is a Certified Holistic Health Coach and co-founder of The Thrive Effect in conjunction with her sister, Christina. Together, Courtney and her sister have built a health coaching business at TheThrive-Effect.com, where they are working to bring health to the masses by using complementary medicine. Courtney has found being a part of the IBD community an important part of her healing story.

"Everyone wants to be part of a community; to be supported, loved and understood. This rings true especially for us, since living with chronic illnesses can feel very isolating at times. One of the things that truly helped me was getting involved in any and all ways that I could. Back when I was first diagnosed, I was involved in the Take Steps walks, running a half marathon with Team Challenge and being open about my journey with IBD (in person and via social media). Now, since my journey has

changed a lot, I am involved within the community by blogging about my holistic perspective on thriving with Crohn's, creating and building my passion project: The Thrive Effect and stepping into my dream of being a holistic health coach for people who live with chronic illness and autoimmune disease and working towards having my own full time coaching practice.

Find a way to get involved, whether it be through talking about your disease and raising awareness, walking/running for a cause, or connecting with other IBDers for a support group. The #1 thing to remember about getting involved is that you don't have to be involved in the same way as everyone else. Finding your own unique way to be a part of the community while using your talents/interests can help you feel supported and connected, while also helping you to incorporate what you love and share something new with other patients into your advocacy efforts... That is truly the best of both worlds!"

As Courtney said, find a way to get involved in the community that resonates with you!

When I was diagnosed, my parents when to Crohn's & Colitis Foundation conferences to educate themselves, and they tried to get me involved, too. They told me about Camp Oasis (a camp for kids with IBD), and whenever they discovered they had a connection to someone else with IBD, they wanted to me to meet with them and talk. That is the opposite of what I wanted! I liked keeping IBD to myself and I hated making a "big deal" out of it.

A few years later, I decided to walk with Take Steps for Crohn's and Colitis, but it was on my decision. Maybe it was my young age of 12 that made me want to have nothing to do with my IBD, but something eventually changed, and doing that first walk sparked a passion to help other people who were standing where I was once.

I look where I stand now and looking in my rearview mirror, it all makes sense. I can see this is how my life was meant to play out. The pain, anger, devastation, and disappointment I have encountered within myself over the years lead me here—to give back to this community. The positive impacts of having Crohn's have outnumbered the negative tenfold. Simply wanting to connect with others online led me to creating a blog, earning an NTP certification, and starting my own nutrition business.

Talk about life changing!

Conclusion

Do you feel it now, the power that is in your hands? I hope you do. I hope you see the many, many, ways in which you influence your own path to health.

Life after diagnosis is complex. It's for sure a journey and not a destination. Diagnosis is just the first step, but utilizing what you know now going forward is absolutely critical. You will go through a trial and error phase where you find out what is the same and what is different from before you were diagnosed. Life won't be completely the same. *And that's okay.*

What matters now is that you use this knowledge and everything that you learn about yourself. I promise, you will come to understand your body very well. I am speaking from over a decade of experience!

You can stumble and fall, but you must always get back up and keep going.

In the words of Alice Walker, *"The most common way people give up their power is by thinking they don't have any."*

In the best of health,

Alexa Federico

Bonuses

Visit this link to get access to bonus material you and download and have access to for life!

http://girlinhealing.com/bookbonuses

Food & Symptom Journal

At Home Must-Haves Checklist

Travel Must-Haves Checklist

Doctor Appointment Checklist

5 under 5 Mindfulness Practices

Medication Tracker Sheet

Real Food Grocery Guide

Be sure to join the companion Facebook group, at http://girlinhealing.com/facebookgroup.

Acknowledgements

Thank you all who have supported Girl in Healing and this book. Every message, comment, and "like" is a boost of encouragement to work for a better life for all with IBD. Thank you to those that have shared their stories with me. Your trust in me is the most prestigious honor I could ask for. You helped create the inspiration for this book.

Thank you to my friends, family, and fellow bloggers who gave me feedback on the content of this book. I would still be pondering the possibilities if it weren't for your decisiveness!

I'd also like to thank my editor, writing mentor, and friend, Dr. Beth Brombosz, whose "Blogger to Author" course streamlined the writing process for me. Thank you for your endless advice and encouragement throughout this journey.

Thank you to my parents, Rob and Sandy who never stopped advocating for me when I couldn't advocate for myself.

Finally, I would like to thank Dr. Emonds, who I literally owe my life to. Thank you for the work you are doing for so many people. The world needs more people like you.

References

1. Ballantyne, S. What is AIP? *The Paleo Mom.* Retrieved from https://www.thepaleomom.com/start-here/the-autoimmune-protocol/

2. What is Crohn's Disease? *Crohn's & Colitis Foundation. Retrieved from* http://www.crohnscolitisfoundation.org/what-are-crohns-and-colitis/what-is-crohns-disease/

3. Understanding Crohn's Disease. *Crohn's & Colitis.* Retrieved from https://www.crohnsandcolitis.com/crohns

4. Irwin M. Suzanne R. Rosenthal IBD Resource Center (IBD Help Center). Aminosalicylates. *Crohn's and & Colitis Foundation.* Retrieved fromhttp://www.crohnscolitisfoundation.org/assets/pdfs/aminosalicylates.pdf

5. Corticosteroids. *Crohn's & Colitis Foundation.* Retrieved from http://www.crohnscolitisfoundation.org/resources/corticosteroids.html

6. Irwin M. Suzanne R. Rosenthal IBD Resource Center (IBD Help Center). Immunomodulators. *Crohn's & Colitis Foundation.* Retrieved from http://www.crohnscolitisfoundation.org/assets/pdfs/immunomodulators.pdf

7. Irwin M. Suzanne R. Rosenthal IBD Resource Center (IBD Help Center). Antibiotics. *Crohn's & Colitis Foundation.* Retrieved from http://www.crohnscolitisfoundation.org/assets/pdfs/antibiotics.pdf

8. D'Haens, G. (2007). Risks and benefits or biologic therapy for inflammatory bowel diseases. *Gut,* 56(5): 725-732. doi: 10.1136/gut.2006.103564.

9. Biologics. *Crohn's & Colitis Foundation.* Retrieved from http://www.crohnscolitisfoundation.org/assets/biologic-therapy.pdf

10. Murat, K., Ibrahim O.K., Ocal, S., Dogan, Z., & Tanoglu, A. (2016). Inefficacy of Triple Therapy and Comparison of Two Different Bismuth-containing Quadruple Regimens as a Firstline Treatment Option for *Heliobacter pylori. Saudi J Gastroenterol,* 22(5): 366-369. doi: 10.4103/1319-3767.191141.

11. Surgery for Crohn's Disease & Ulcerative Colitis. *Crohn's & Colitis Foundation.* Retrieved from http://www.crohnscolitisfoundation.org/resources/surgery-for-crohns-uc.html

12. Crohn's Treatments. *Crohn's & Coltiis.* Retrieved from https://www.crohnsandcolitis.com/crohns/disease-treatment

13. Colectomy *Surgical Removal of the Colon. American College of Surgeons.* Retrieved from https://www.facs.org/~/media/files/education/patie nt%20ed/2015%20colectomy%20brochure%20fina l.ashx

14. Lopez, J., Grinspan, A. (2016). Fecal Microbiota Transplantation for Inflammatory Bowel Disase. *Gastroenterol Hepatol (N Y),* 12(6): 374-379.

15. Carrera-Bastos, P., Fontes-Villalba, M., O'Keefe, J.H., Lindeberg, & S., Cordain, L. (2011). The western diet and lifestyle and diseases of civilization. *Research Reports in Clinical Cardiology,* 2, 15-35. doi: 10.2147/RRCC.S16919.

16. Gradisar, M., Wolfson, A. R., Harvey, A. G., Hale, L., Rosenberg, R., & Czeisler, C. A. (2013). The Sleep and Technology Use of Americans: Findings from the National Sleep Foundation's 2011 Sleep in America Poll. *Journal of Clinical Sleep Medicine : JCSM : Official Publication of the American Academy of Sleep Medicine,* 9(12), 1291–1299. doi: 10.5664/jcsm.3272.

17. Keefer, L., Keshavarzian, A., & Mutlu, E. (2008). Reconsidering the methodology of "stress" research in inflammatory bowel disease. *Journal of Crohn's and Colitis,* 2(3), 193-201. doi: 10.1016/j.crohns.2008.01.002.

18. Ng, V., Millard, W., Lebrun, C., & Howard, J. (2006). Exercise and Crohn's Disease: Speculations on Potential Benefits. *Canadian*

Journal of Gastroenterology, 20(10), 657-660. doi: 10.1155/2006/462495.

19. Sonnenberg, A. (1990). Occupational distribution of inflammatory bowel disease among German employees. *Gut,* 31, 1037-1040.

20. Alkouri, R.H., Hashmi, H., Baker, R.D., Gelfond, D., & Baker, S.S. (2013). Vitamin and Mineral Status in Patients With Inflammatory Bowel Disease. *Journal of Pediatric Gastroenterology and Nutrition,* 56(1), 89-92. doi: 10.1097/MPG.0b013e31826a105d.

21. Issokson, K. (2017). Common Micronutrient Deficiencies in IBD. *Crohn's & Colitis Foundation.* Retrieved from http://www.crohnscolitisfoundation.org/science-and-professionals/nutrition-resource-/micronutrient-deficiency-fact.pdf.

22. Rogler, G., & Vavricka, S. (2014). Anemia in Inflammatory Bowel Disease: An Under-Estimated Problem? *Frontiers in Medicine,* 1, 58. foi: 10.3389/fmed.2014.00058.

23. Langmead, L. et al. (2004). Randomized, double-blind, placebo-controlled trial of oral aloe vera gel for active ulcerative colitis. Alimentary Pharmacological Therapies, 19, 739-747.

24. Konijeti, G.G. et al. (2017). Efficacy of the Autoimmune Protocol Diet for Inflammatory Bowel Disease. Inflammatory Bowel Diseases, doi:

10.1097/MIB.0000000000001221.

25. Stenson, W.F.D. et al. (1992). Dietary supplementation with fish oil in ulcerative colitis. Annals of Internal Medicine, 116(8), 609-614.

26. Joseph, A.J. et al. (2009). 25(OH) vitamin D levels in Crohn's disease: association with sun exposure & disease activity. Indian Journal of Medical Research, 130, 133-137.

27. Ammon, H.P.T. (2010). Modulation of the immune system by Boswellia serrata extracts and boswellic acids. Phytomedicine, 17Omer et al., 2007, 862-867.

28. Ammon, H.P. (2016). Boswellic Acids and Their Role in Chronic Inflammatory Diseases. Advanced in Experimental Medicine and Biology, 928, 291-327.

29. Gerhardt, H. et al. (2011). [Therapy of active Crohn disease with Boswellia serrata extract H 15].[Article in German]. Z Gastroenterol, 39(1), 11-17.

30. Pellegrini, L. et al. (2016). Managing ulcerative colitis in remission phase: usefulness of Casperome®, an innovative lecithin-based delivery system of Boswellia serrata extract. European Reviews in Medical Pharmacological Science, 20(12), 2695-2700.

31. Lachenmeier, D.W. (2010). Letter to the Editor: Wormwood (Artemisia absinthium L.)—A curious plant with both neurotoxic and neuroprotective properties? Journal of Ethnopharmacology, 131(1), 224-227.

32. Van Dullemen, H.M. et al. (1995). Treatment of Crohn's disease with anti-tumour necrosis factor chimeric antibody (cA2). Gastroenterology, 109, 129-135.

33. Omer, B. et al. (2007). Steroid-sparing effect of wormwood (Artemisia absinthium) in Crohn's disease: A double-blind placebo-controlled study. Phytomedicine, 14(2-3), 87-95.

34. Krebs, S. et al. (2010). Wormwood (Artemisia absinthium) suppresses tumour necrosis factor alpha and accelerates healing in patients with Crohn's disease - A controlled clinical trial. Phytomedicine, 17(5), 305-309. doi: 10.1016/j.phymed.2009.10.013.

35. Kocaadam, B., & Sanlier, N. (2017). Curcumin, an active component of turmeric (Curcuma longa), and its effects on health. Critical Reviews in Food Science and Nutrition, 57(13), 2889-2895. http://dx.doi.org.uws.idm.oclc.org/10.1080/104083 98.2015.1077195

36. Holt, P.R., Katz, S., & Kirshoff, R. (2005). Curcumin therapy in inflammatory bowel disease: A pilot study. Digestive Diseases and Sciences,

50(11), 2191-2193.

37. Lang, A. et al. (2015). Curcumin in Combination With Mesalamine Induces Remission in Patients With Mild-to-Moderate Ulcerative Colitis in a Randomized Controlled Trial. Clinical Gastroenterology and Hepatology, 13(8), 1444-1440. doi: 10.1016/j.cgh.2015.02.019.

38. Ghosh, S.S. et al. (2014). Oral supplementation with non-absorbable antibiotics or curcumin attenuates western diet-induced atherosclerosis and glucose intolerance in LDLR-/- mice--role of intestinal permeability and macrophage activation. PLoS One, 9(9), e108577. doi: 10.1371/journal.pone.0108577.

39. Sabeh, F. et al. (1996). Isozymes of superoxide dismutase from Aloe vera. Enzyme Protein, 49(4), 212-221.

40. t'Hart, L.A. et al. (1989). An anti-complementary polysaccharide with immunological adjuvant activity from the leaf parenchyma gel of Aloe vera. Planta Medicine, 55(6), 509-512.

41. Sahl, B. et al. (2003). Curcumin attenuates DNB-induced murine colitis. Gastrointestinal and Liver Physiology, 285(1), G235-G243 doi: 10.1152/ajpgi.00449.2002.

42. Spanier, G. et al. (2008). Resveratrol reduces endothelial oxidative stress by modulating the gene expression of superoxide dismutase 1 (SOD1),

glutathione peroxidase 1 (GPx1) and NADPH oxidase subunit (Nox4). Phytochemistry, 69(8), 1732-1738.

43. Yao, J. et al. (2010). Anti-oxidant effects of resveratrol on mice with DSS-induced ulcerative colitis. Archives of Medical Research, 41(4), 288-294.

44. Sánchez-Fidalgo, S. et al. (2010). Dietary supplementation of resveratrol attenuates chronic colonic inflammation in mice. Asian Pacific Journal of Clinical Nutrition, 19(1), 142-150.

45. Frolkis, A. et al. (2013). Environment and the inflammatory bowel diseases. *Canadian Journal of Gastroenterology,* 27(3), e-18-e24.

46. Brodin, P. et al. (2015). Variation in the human immune system is largely driven by non-heritable influences. *Cell,* 160, 37-47.

47. Mach, T., & Szczeklik, K. (2017). Crohn's Disease and Its Oral Manifestations. *Journal of Gastroenterology, Hepatology, and Endoscopy,* 2(2), 1012.

48. de Punder, K., & Pruimboom, L. (2013). The Dietary Intake of Wheat and other Cereal Grains and Their Role in Inflammation. *Nutrients,* 5(3), 771-787. doi: 10.3390/nu5030771.

49. Vasconcelos, I.M., & Oliveira, J.T.A. (2004). Antinutritional properties of plant lectins. *Science*

Direct, 4(15), 385-403.

50. Fasano, A. (2012). Zonulin, regulation of tight junctions, and autoimmune diseases. *Annals of the New York Academy of Sciences,* 1258(1), 25-33. doi: 10.1111/j.1749-6632.2012.06538.x

51. Herfarth, H.H., Martin, C.F., Sandler, R.S., Kappelman, M.D., & Long, M.D. (2014). Prevalence of a gluten free diet and improvement of clinical symptoms with inflammatory bowel diseases. *Inflammatory Bowel Diseases,* 20(7), 1194-1197. doi: 10.1097/MIB.0000000000000077.

52. Konijeti, G.G., et al. (2017) Efficacy of the Autoimmune Protocol Diet for Inflammatory Bowel Disease. *Inflammatory Bowel Diseases,* 23(11), 2054-2060. doi: 10.1097/MIB.0000000000001221.

53. Gorad, D.A., et al. (1993). Initial response and subsequent course of Crohn's disease treated with elemental diet or prednisolone. *Gut,* 34, 1198-1202. doi: 10.1136/gut.34.9.1198.

About the Author

Alexa Federico is an author and blogger at her website Girl in Healing, a hub dedicated to providing recipes and resources to help people with IBD. She was diagnosed with Crohn's when she was 12 years old and has tested out numerous conventional and alternative therapies to help her heal. Alexa was motivated to write this book based on a lack of "first steps" for people diagnosed with Crohn's and colitis. Her own health journey sparked a fire in her to learn and teach what real nutrition looks like and the role it plays in healing. She is a practicing Nutritional Therapy Practitioner and an AIP Certified Health Coach specializing in digestion and autoimmunity and works with clients remotely.

Made in the USA
Lexington, KY
24 May 2018